Self-determined Dying

Manual for a rational Suicide

Method

"Plastic bag and sleeping pills"

Self-determined Dying
Manual for a rational Suicide
Method "Plastic bag and sleeping pills"

First published April 2020

Jessica Düber
Orleansstraße 22
31135 Hildesheim

Printversion by
Amazon Media EU S.à r.l., 5 Rue Plaetis,
L-2338 Luxembourg

ISBN 9798637388042

Foreword

On 26.02.2020, the German Federal Constitutional Court declared the controversial paragraph 217 of the German Penal Code to be null and void. The right to self-determination concerning one's own death was thus confirmed. The verdict states that the right to die self-determined includes the freedom to take one's own life. It explicitly states that this right to self-determination is due to every person - even without the presence of illness. In order to put this right into practice, professional help must from now on be available to people. Of course, these aids should be based on certain rules and criteria that enable a responsible implementation of the judgement. What exactly the implementation will look like now will become apparent in the next months.

However, I do not believe that this positive development should lead us to rely solely on the implementation of policy. I still think it is important to familiarise oneself with the possibilities for rational suicide. In my opinion, a greater number of options and thus an increase in personal freedom of choice is always desirable.

In 2017 I wrote the book " Self-determined Dying - Manual for a rational suicide". Meanwhile there are also updated versions of the two most important and reliable methods "Chloroquine" and "Helium". In the 2017 handbook I wanted to present possibilities for which there was already a minimum amount of empirical data and which - at that time I was guided by the "Sesarid Criteria" formulated by Boudewijn Chabot (see Chabot, Boudewijn: Dignified Dying, 2017; p.85ff) - meet the requirements of a "peaceful dying".

In the meantime, my criteria for introducing possibilities of rational suicide have changed. I don't want to make only proven recommendations, but rather point out options and bring them into the public discussion. I am looking forward to a possible exchange of ideas about possible methodological improvements. Based on such an attitude, I have recently written a small handbook on the method "Carotid Artery". This was prompted by numerous inquiries from readers who had heard or read about certain methods and now wanted to know "more details". I would like these handouts to be understood as a way to deal with the advantages and disadvantages of a method on a theoretical level - if, on the other hand, you are looking for guidance on an established and empirically reliable method, I would rather recommend the "Helium" or "Chloroquine" methods.

In this small handbook the method "plastic bag with sleeping pills" is presented. One advantage of the method is that the necessary utensils are comparatively easy to obtain. For methods that use chloroquine or noble gases, it is always a prerequisite that the required materials have either already been procured beforehand or that there are still procurement possibilities in case of a wish to die. Recently there have been difficulties in obtaining chloroquine from pharmacies - we need to look further into how chloroquine can be obtained in the future. The method described here also requires drugs - but these are sleeping pills, and there are no major hurdles to obtaining them. One could therefore consider the method "plastic bag with sleeping pills" as a kind of "emergency plan" and familiarize oneself with it in order to have an alternative for self-determined dying in a case where other methods are no longer feasible.

Basic principle of the method

It is an old and quite well-known method: a plastic bag is pulled over the head and fastened at the neck with a comfortable but tight-fitting elastic band. In the closed bag the oxygen is used up by breathing; this lack of oxygen finally leads to brain death. In addition, exhalation causes an increase in carbon dioxide inside the bag and thus also leads to carbon dioxide poisoning. By taking sleeping pills beforehand, the person willing to die is already in a deep unconsciousness during this process; negative reactions to the increasing carbon dioxide content inside the bag are thus prevented.

The method is basically simple and it does not require much effort to obtain the necessary utensils; however, there are a few things to consider that are elementary for a successful implementation. There are numerous, partly insufficient descriptions and conclusions for implementation. A very good discussion of the method can be found in the book by Chris Docker (see Docker, Chris, 2015: Five Last Acts - The Exit Path. 2015 edition with additional material; 301-324 and 452-460). Here first of all the "Basics":

- An antiemetic (drug that is effective against nausea and vomiting) is taken some time before the planned execution of self-determined dying

- A large (!) plastic bag is pulled over the head. It is

closed at the neck with a rubber band previously placed around the neck by pushing the ends of the bag under the rubber band. In order to prevent the bag from touching the face directly, a wide-brimmed (sun) hat can be worn under the plastic bag. The bag is completely filled with air (by swiveling it through the room) before it is attached under the elastic band

- Before the bag is pulled over the head in the described manner, sleeping pills are taken

- Death occurs due to a lack of oxygen and poisoning by CO2. Since the person is already in a deep sleep before the oxygen is used up and the CO2 content in the bag is so high that the body may react with an alarm, death finally occurs without any unpleasant experiences for the person willing to die

The air that we "normally" breathe is a mixture of the two gases oxygen (approx. 21%) and nitrogen (approx. 78%). It also contains small amounts of argon, carbon dioxide and traces of other gases. In simple terms, the human body needs oxygen and produces carbon dioxide (CO_2) as a waste product which is exhaled again. The cause of death in the method described here is asphyxia, i.e. an undersupply of oxygen to the body, which eventually leads to death, and poisoning by CO2. The plastic bag is initially filled with air containing oxygen. As you breathe, the oxygen content in the bag decreases. At the same time, the amount of CO2 in the bag increases, as CO2 is exhaled as a "waste product".

The human body reacts not particularly sensitive to a drop in the concentration of vital oxygen in the air we breathe. What the human body does react very sensitively to, however, in contrast to a drop in the concentration of oxygen in the air we breathe, is the increase in carbon dioxide in the air we breathe. With the method of wanting to induce asphyxiation death by simply putting a plastic bag over the head and fastening it, in which an increased concentration of CO^2 from the exhaled air is produced, the person willing to die would at some point try in panic to tear the plastic bag off his head. This fact makes it necessary to carry out the method with a previous intake of sleeping pills.

I have already pointed out in earlier publications (e.g. the comments on the helium method) that even when using a plastic bag in combination with non-lethal sleeping pills, there is still the risk that the bag is torn from the head by involuntary, hectic movements - and this is when the sleeping pills do not have enough time to develop their full effect before the CO2 content inside the bag has risen to such an extent that the body reacts with an alarm.

Another reason for this reaction would also be that the chosen medication is basically not able to produce a sufficiently deep sleep (for example, when using over-the-counter sleeping pills or other unsuitable sedatives).

However, it is very important to choose a sufficiently large plastic bag. If the plastic bag has been chosen to be sufficiently large, the sleeping pills that have been taken before the bag was pulled over the head will have sufficient time to take effect. The aim is to achieve a deep sleep in which unconscious, reflex-like actions are no longer possible.

There are different stages of sleep - from light sleep to deep unconsciousness. For example, if during normal night sleep the blanket covers a person's face and interferes with breathing, the person will unconsciously make a hand movement to push the blanket away. However, there are also stages of sleep (for example, after taking a large dose of suitable sleeping pills) where these reflex-like reactions no longer occur. A very deep sleep is therefore necessary to ensure that you do not reflexively pull the bag off your head when the CO_2 content inside the plastic bag increases. Even after taking a high overdose of suitable sleeping pills, it takes some time before the sleep is sufficiently deep.

The method can be performed both lying down and sitting. I would prefer the lying position for this method, as no further precautions for fixing the body are necessary, apart from the fact that the head can be cushioned a little bit at the side with pillows. If the method is to be carried out while sitting (e.g. in an armchair), it is important to fix the body completely before. It is possible, for example, to fix the upper body with a yoga belt or similar directly to an armchair with a high backrest. This is to prevent the body from falling forward or to the side after the sleeping pills have taken effect and to prevent the plastic bag on the head from slipping and to prevent the ends of the bag from being pulled out from under the elastic band.

Below follows a description of the other details to be observed.

The plastic bag

As described above, it is of absolute importance that the bag is sufficiently large. The bag should allow for free breathing for about 50 minutes after being placed on the head to give the sedatives that have been taken enough time to produce a deep sleep. With this method, the larger the bag, the better (this is different with the helium method, for example). Again, the bigger the bag, the more difficult it is to handle.

To be able to estimate the size, however, one does not necessarily have to calculate. In the above-mentioned publication, Docker suggests, for example, that you check the size by sitting in an armchair and putting the bag on to try it out. The bag is filled with air beforehand by swivelling it briefly through the air. The ends of the bag are placed under a rubber band (or several rubber bands) that fits tightly around the neck. If the other end (the closed end) of the bag then reaches about to the lap when sitting upright, the size is fine. When using this method, also remember that the bag will not stand up (as is the case with the helium method, for example). Since the bag is only filled with "normal" air from the room, it has no buoyancy or the like; it will therefore "look for" a supporting surface. By the way - do not be afraid of such experiments - they are not dangerous and even very important. I will go into more detail below about the need to rehearse the procedure. In addition to the possibility of testing the correct size of a bag in the way described, you can also use a litre indication of about 240l capacity as a reference point for your purchase. This is a common size for bin liners of strong quality. Unfortunately these extra strong bin liners are mainly offered in opaque design. I rather recommend to choose a transparent bag - but this is only for aesthetic reasons and because of the idea that it is still possible to look out of a transparent bag. For example, you could, if you wish, look out of the window into the sky or into nature until the sleeping pills take effect, or look at a beautiful bouquet of flowers that you have placed near the position you have chosen for your dying.

When searching for transparent bags, you can also use the dimensions given as a guide. A good size would be about 150cm x 100cm.

With vacuum bags, which often have these dimensions, it is important to ensure that these are models that are only deflated by rolling them up, otherwise the holes intended for the suction are often in the middle of the bag, which represents an undesirable risk of leakage. The closures of the vacuum bags (the sealing) must be cut off in order to be able to put the bag under the rubber band at the neck. This must be taken into account when choosing the size.

With regard to strength, it is important to choose a material that is not too thin. On the other hand, as the strength of the material increases, it also becomes more difficult to insert the bag under the elastic in order to fasten it securely and airtight. It is also possible to put two bags inside each other and then fill the inner bag with air by swivelling. This double-layered use would provide greater security with regard to the tightness of the bag. It may be a little surprising - but by no means all plastic bags are airtight over a long period of time. Thus, it can be useful to consider the properties of the plastic used in advance - some plastics are more permeable to air than others, for example. The thinner and cheaper the plastic is, the more air permeable it will be - especially if airtightness is not necessary for the original purpose of the bag (bin liners etc.) one should critically check whether the airtightness of the material is sufficient for the planned project. It is important that the bag used does not allow oxygen from the outside to pass through the material, as this would endanger the success of your plan. The marking of the plastic used may provide information about its physical properties.

Fastening the bag with an elastic band

In my descriptions of the helium method I have included instructions for manufacturing a so-called ExitBag. It is a plastic bag with an integrated elastic band at the hem, which allows you to put the bag on quickly and comfortably and which holds the bag securely but loosely around your neck. I do not recommend such a production for the method "plastic bag with sleeping pills". With the helium method, the rubber band only has the task of preventing the helium-filled bag from flying away. Helium is lighter than air and would, as known from helium balloons, rise into the air. The fact that the ExitBag does not fit snugly around the neck is also desirable here, since the inflowing helium permanently displaces the exhaled CO_2 through the not completely sealing points around the neck. With the method "plastic bag with sleeping pills" on the other hand, the function of the rubber band is quite different.

The plastic bag does not need to be secured against flying away, as it is only filled with room air. No gas needs to be displaced from the bag - above all, no fresh oxygen should be able to enter the bag from the ambient air, as the continuous consumption of the oxygen inside the bag is what we intend and want to achieve. It is therefore important that the bag fits tightly around the neck and that there are no leaks. This is best achieved by fitting one elastic band (for safety's sake there can be several elastic bands) to the neck so that it fits tightly. However, it should not cut in or be uncomfortable. To avoid unpleasant sensations, do not let the rubber band run over the larynx, but over or under it. Suitable for example is a 5mm wide elastic braid that has been adapted to your own neck by means of a secure knot (it is advisable to use several elastics for such a small thickness) or an elastic braid in larger width, which has been sewn fitting securely to the neck circumference.

The ends of the bag are then placed under this elastic band. Insert the bag generously under the elastic band so that the ends cannot accidentally slip out from under the elastic band. The ends should protrude at least 20cm under the rubber band; even if the ends protrude more under the rubber band, this is not a problem (as long as the total available volume of the bag is large enough). While trying and practicing the method, you will find out how the thickness of the material of the bag also affects the possibility of a tight and, if possible, wrinkle-free attachment under the rubber band. This practising is extremely important to get a feeling for how the bag can be fastened well and airtightly to the neck by means of rubber band.

The sleeping pills

Sleeping pills are necessary to ensure a deep sleep and thus suppress reflex reactions to the increasing carbon dioxide content inside the bag. The sleeping pills themselves are not lethal but only sleep-inducing. There are several sleeping pills that can be used - the important thing is that they induce a deep sleep for you personally. It can vary from person to person which sleeping pills work well.

There are sleeping pills that are available without a prescription. Over-the-counter sleeping pills usually contain an antihistamine; either diphenhydramine or doxylamine. Neither of these substances is used as an antihistamine any more, as there are now active ingredients available that can be used to treat allergic reactions more specifically and without side effects. However, the active substances are still used as sleeping pills due to their sedative component. I would strongly advise against this type of sleeping pill for the "plastic bag and sleeping pills" method; they are not particularly potent sleep promoters and an overdose will most likely cause very unpleasant side effects. One mistake that often leads to failure with the "plastic bag with sleeping pills" method is to choose unsuitable sleeping pills.

It is safer to use sleeping pills that are available only on prescription. One possibility would be benzodiazepines. Benzodiazepines are drugs commonly called sleeping pills or tranquillisers. The benzodiazepine subgroup includes many different drugs. The spectrum of action of the individual active ingredients ranges from sleep-inducing to anxiety-relieving, antispasmodic, muscle-relaxing, calming, mood-lifting and euphoric. Benzodiazepines are usually non-fatal even in high overdoses.

Benzodiazepines have a high potential for addiction, so doctors have now switched to prescribing sleeping pills from the group known as "Z-drugs". Although these are now thought to have a similarly high dependence potential to benzodiazepines, they are currently the most commonly prescribed sleeping pills in Europe and the USA. There are slight pharmacodynamic differences between benzodiazepines and Z-drugs; they differ structurally but bind to the same receptors and have a similar spectrum of action. The muscle-relaxing and antispasmodic effects of Z-drugs are less than those of benzodiazepines. Z-drugs can also be used to induce deep sleep; care should be taken when choosing a drug to ensure that it has a long half-life. I recommend the use of benzodiazepines, as there is already a lot of experience of successful self-managed dying for this use; the best would be diezepam, a benzodiazepine that works for a long time and can be prescribed for sleep disorders. But since it is easier to get Z-substances prescribed, you can also use Zopiclon or Zolpidem, for example. But please be sure to follow the instructions I give below to determine the necessary amount.

Those who know my manual on the chloroquine method may remember that I recommend the use of diazepam in liquid form. This does not apply to the method "plastic bag with sleeping pills". The effect may set in so quickly that it is no longer possible to place and fix the bag correctly. With the chloroquine method, on the other hand, the last step is to take the diazepam drops - no further action is required and falling asleep immediately does not pose any problems and is even desirable. For the method "plastic bag with sleeping pills" I recommend the use of tablets instead of drops. Please note that crushed or powdered tablets have a faster onset of action than intact tablets.

But in which dose should one take the sleeping pill one has opted for or which is available to one? As there are theoretically a lot of drugs that can be used, I do not want to give any dosage information. I suggest that you first familiarize yourself with the package insert and check which dose is recommended for the intended purpose (treatment of sleep disorders).

Then test the effect of this recommended dose yourself. For this test you should choose a day when you have nothing else to do. Ideally you should start in the morning - not in the evening. It is not particularly meaningful if you "test" sleeping pills in the evening - in a situation where you might have fallen asleep anyway. So make yourself comfortable in bed in the morning with a book or magazine. Then take the dose of the sleeping pills recommended in the package leaflet. Leave the curtains open so that the room is bright and do not take any precautions that have anything to do with your usual "sleeping rituals". You want to find out if the sleeping pill is so potent that it will cause you to sleep in a situation where you would not normally sleep.

If you can, try to observe how long it takes for the sleeping pill to put you to sleep. It also matters how long you slept. If the dose recommended in the package leaflet did not force you to sleep for about seven hours, you should repeat the test after a few days and increase the dose. When you have finally found out what dose is sufficient for you to produce a deep sleep of about seven hours, multiply this number of tablets by a factor of 15 - and then take this number of tablets to induce a deep sleep during the planned suicide.

Taking an antiemetic

An antiemetic is a drug that works against nausea and vomiting. In order to achieve a sufficiently deep sleep, the sleeping pills must be given in high doses. The body might react to this kind of poisoning with vomiting. However, if the sleeping pills taken, or part of them, are vomited, it is likely that the amount of active ingredient still present in the body is not sufficient to produce a sufficiently deep sleep. The body may then react to the increasing CO_2 content of the air inside the bag, and the person willing to die may tear the bag off his head by reflexive movements.

Vomiting in general (also with other methods) is a frequent cause of failure of a suicide attempt and it can be effectively prevented by taking an antiemetic. The drug of first choice for preventing vomiting is the active ingredient metoclopramide (MCP). Drops are preferable to tablets; absorption is more reliable. If only tablets are available, these can of course also be used. The active ingredient Domperidone (trade names e.g. Domidon, Motilium) can also be used. Here is an exemplary intake schedule for MCP:

24 hours before the suicide 10mg MCP and
16 hours before the suicide 10mg MCP and
8 hours before the suicide 10mg MCP and
45 minutes before the suicide 10mg MCP

Prevent early detection

If one has taken note of all the information listed so far, which is important for the planning of the suicide, it is important to make provision for the immediate time after suicide as well. It is undesirable to be found at a time when death has not yet arrived and life-saving measures may be initiated. This means that the situation should be prepared in such a way that untimely discovery by uninformed persons does not take place. Since situations can not be planned one hundred percent, it is also advisable to create or have created a patient's provision and to position this within sight bevor self-determined dying is executed. In a patient's provision, for example, you can state that you do not want any life-saving measures. This disposition is theoretically legally binding once the patient's provision has been signed and dated. However, it is relatively likely that incoming first-aiders, whether professional helpers or lay people, feel it is their job to save lives and act accordingly. Thus, creating a situation where you are not found early would be the most appropriate.

The following period should be allowed for dying with the "plastic bag and sleeping pill" method: Duration for which the selected size of the plastic bag provides a supply of oxygen, i.e. one can continue to breathe while the sleeping pills taken are taking effect, plus approx. 30 minutes. If you can ensure privacy for about 2 hours, you are on the safe side with the bag size discussed above.

Procurement

The following substances are needed:

- Metoclopramide
- Sleeping Pills (e.g. Diazepam, Zopiclon, Zolpidem)

Procurement of metoclopramide

Metoclopramide is a prescription medicine for nausea and vomiting that can be prescribed without major hurdles by a family doctor. So you can just go to a family doctor and describe the symptoms (for example, migraine-related nausea). It may be helpful to tell the doctor that you have previously been prescribed MCP drops and have tolerated them well. If necessary, familiarize yourself with the package leaflet (can be accessed online) to be able to argue accordingly.

If you do not want to go to the doctor for a prescription, you can order Metoclopramide (only in tablet form, which is okay as well) here:

https://www.dokteronline.com/de/mcp?sqr=mcp&

"Dokteronline" is a so-called online clinic. These online clinics offer medical advice from independent EU physicians and issue prescriptions for medications without actually seeing the patient. First of all, you select for which drug you would like to have a prescription and then fill in a questionnaire. This questionnaire will then be evaluated by a physician cooperating with the clinic and the issue of the prescription will either be approved (if the answers to the questionnaire do not indicate any risk factors for taking the drug) or refused. For opioid analgesics there is also a maximum order quantity in a given period. You can also choose whether you want to receive only the prescription or whether the online clinic should forward the prescription to a mail order pharmacy, which then sends the drug directly to your home. Those who prefer to receive only the prescription and to pick up the drug in the pharmacy of his confidence will be sent a private prescription whose redemption in a pharmacy does not cause any difficulties. Due to the so-called patient mobility directive, an adaptation in the European legislation, it is now possible for patients to be treated at their own choice in other European countries. Generally speaking, it is legitimate to use services in the health sector across borders, and thus prescriptions from other EU countries can be redeemed everywhere. However, prescriptions from other EU countries are always considered as private prescriptions and the medication must therefore be paid by yourself.

Incidentally, MCP drops are part of many private medicine cupboards. Possibly worthwhile for obtaining MCP could therefore be inquiries in the circle of acquaintances and friends.

Procurement of sleeping pills

Benzodiazepines or Z-Drugs cannot be obtained through an online clinic.

So one way to get these substances is to go to a doctor and report symptoms that are usually treated with the drug. You could report persistent sleep disorders that you have already tried to alleviate with various improvements in lifestyle and sleep hygiene. However, benzodiazepines or Z-drugs are not drugs that treat the cause of a disorder, they relieve symptoms. So it might be promising if it is reported that work is already going on to treat the cause of the problem (e.g. you already have an appointment with a psychotherapist because of your sleep problems, but it is far in the future) and now you need a drug to be able to "get through" certain situations before you start treatment. It may help if you report that you are currently facing professional events for which you need to be well rested. It might also help if you report that you have had an upsetting event that has thrown you off track to such an extent that you now need a temporary sleeping pill to get through the next period and to be able to fall asleep (for example, a separation, a death, etc.). If you like it less dramatic, you can also report that you are going on holiday with your partner where you do not have two separate bedrooms as usual - and since your partner snores a lot, you would like to have sleeping pills so that you can have a restful sleep on holiday. This procedure may not lead to immediate success. The doctor may initially recommend a drug that is not potent enough for our purposes. You may also be given a prescription for the basically usable Zopiclon. You should then first go home with the prescription and visit the doctor again after a certain time if you have the desire to use another substance, for example a benzodiazepine. At this next appointment, it can be reported that the prescribed medication was not well tolerated, but the corresponding condition persists, so the doctor will prescribe another medication. This procedure can be repeated until you receive a prescription for the desired sleeping pills. Of course, it is also possible to tell the doctor about your symptoms and to point out that you have already been prescribed the desired medication in the past and that your experience with it has been very good. This may speed up the desired prescription.

Another source of supply would be friends and relatives, possibly also a circle of interested people who exchange medication among themselves. If people are prescribed medication because they suffer from a certain disease or condition, they often do not take the prescribed medication exactly in the prescribed dose. Sometimes the dose is increased, sometimes the dose is undercut or other medication is used in addition, so that there can be an accumulated surplus of medication that can be used for self-determined dying. Another theoretically conceivable possibility (I would like to emphasize that I am not suggesting any illegal actions here) would be the falsification of private prescriptions.

The black market also offers opportunities for purchase,

whereby buying on the real black market requires connections that perhaps only a few people have or wish to make.

However, the increasing shift of real markets into the digital world does not stop at the black markets or grey markets (so-called "grey goods" here are substances that were obtained as drugs from originally legal treatments or prescriptions), and so the increase in digital distribution in this area also ensures that black or grey market goods such as drugs or prescription drugs can now be comfortably ordered from the couch at home. The use of the so-called darknet markets (see Wikipedia – article) requires an understanding of the procedures (install certain browsers, get the currency Bitcoins etc.), but is ultimately manageable for anyone with some common sense. If, after receiving drugs, one is unsure whether the substance obtained really corresponds to the desired one, it is possible to have a chemical analysis of the substance carried out. In a suitable laboratory, however, this is relatively expensive for private individuals. The quantitative analysis (how much of a certain active ingredient does the substance contain) is even more complex than the qualitative analysis (does the substance contain a certain active ingredient), so that when buying on the so-called black or grey market (both in the "real world" and online), a residual risk remains with regard to the active ingredient and purity content of the substances. You can also ask a pharmacy to examine the substance but pharmacies are not obliged to analyse substances, so they can refuse this request.

The problem that consumers of illegal substances have no knowledge of the ingredients and are therefore in an unsafe and dangerous situation is of course well known. In the field of accepting drug work, projects for "drug checking" have therefore been developed in the past. Drug Checking offers people the opportunity to have the substances they want to consume chemically analysed and thus reduce the risks associated with consumption (for example, through contamination or unusual high concentrations of active substances).

Theoretically, it would therefore be conceivable to have the substances acquired in the "Darknet" chemically analysed by a Drug Checking unit. However, most of the centres are located outside Germany. In countries such as Spain, Switzerland, Austria and the Netherlands, the harm-reducing approach of drug checking has been established and proven for decades. In Germany, implementation has been difficult in the past. A drug checking project is now to be implemented in Berlin in 2020, but the exact dates for the beginning of this offer have not yet been fixed.

Despite these very positive developments and possibilities it may not be a very attractive idea for some people to travel around with substances acquired in the " Darknet " in order to have them analysed somewhere. Therefore, I would like to introduce a very ambitious Spanish project that offers the possibility to send in substances for analysis by postal mail: Energy Control from Barcelona.

Energy Control is a project to reduce the risks associated with the use of so-called party drugs, which began in

Barcelona in 1997. Since 1999 Energy Control has been offering drug checking. Since 2014 the chemical analysis of substances is also offered internationally and samples can be sent by postal service. With this service Energy Control explicitly addresses users outside Spain. The analytical techniques used allow both qualitative and quantitative analysis of substances. The service offered is anonymous and confidential. Energy Control works in accordance with strict data protection regulations. The data collected may be used for research purposes; however, no personal information about you will be used for this purpose. The communication regarding the test results is done by email, so anonymity is also possible. Energy Control also explicitly points out the possibilities of encrypted communication. Payment for services is possible by bank transfer, Paypal or Bitcoin. After arrival of the samples in the laboratory, it takes between one and three weeks until a result is available and sent to you by email. Under the following link Energy Control has compiled all relevant information in English:

https://energycontrol-international.org/

If you want to send in a sample, simply use the following link:

https://energycontrol-international.org/drug-testing-service/submitting-a-sample/

Storage

Anyone who finally has procured all the necessary drugs may be interested in keeping them for the longest possible period of time without losing their effectiveness (especially in the event that the drugs have been provided to prepare for the future). A use-by date is always specified on the packaging of a drug. The manufacturer guarantees that the substance is effective *at least* until this date if stored appropriately. Most drugs have a guaranteed shelf life of about four to five years from the date of manufacture. However, it can be assumed that medicines will not show any reduction in effectiveness under favorable storage conditions for at least ten years from the date of manufacture. An optimal storage place for drugs would be a uniformly cool, dark place. An unheated (but necessarily frost-free) room in the house (for example a bedroom) is well suited. At this location, the drugs should be stored in their original packaging and additionally be packed in airtight containers (for example a glass with a screw-cap or a "Tupperbox"). Optionally, one or more small sachets of silica gel (silica gel is being used as a desiccant and traded in small sachets) may be placed in the airtight container. Silica gel is highly moisture absorbent and can absorb up to 40% of moisture of its own weight. The need to protect the substances from moisture is, of course, mainly related to the case where one has medication in tablet form. MCP drops, for example, do not need to be protected from moisture. It is important to protect other people from accidental or unauthorized access to the substances. It would therefore be ideal to store the airtight container (the glass with a screw-cap or the Tupperbox) additionally in a lockable cassette or box. Storage in the refrigerator offers no advantages and is unnecessary. It also increases the risk of accidental or unauthorized access by others.

Exact schedule

To conclude, I would like to present a very concrete schedule, which you can use as a guide in your preparations.

Of course, it starts with getting the necessary items. I recommend not to do this only when you have an actual need, but to prepare and store a box with all materials in advance. Early preparation is also important because I strongly recommend that you practice with the materials extensively. I will explain this further below. But first of all your " shopping list":

You need:

- A large plastic bag
  (Information on material and size can be found above)

- Several rubber bands
  (Information on the required quality can be found above)

- Sleeping pills
  (Above, I have described, which substances are suitable, how you can find out the right amount for yourself, what are the possibilities of procurement and how the drugs are stored optimally)

- An antiemetic
  (Above, I have shown which substances can be used, how the antiemetic is dosed, what possibilities there are for procuring it and how the drugs are optimally stored)

- Optionally you can also provide a (sun) - hat with a wide brim. You will notice while practicing if it is more comfortable for you to wear a hat during the performance. The wide brim of the hat is to prevent the plastic bag from sinking down onto your face (this can happen especially when lying down) and thus cause an unpleasant feeling

When you have got all the necessary items, you should practice the whole procedure a few times. Of course, you should not take any sleeping pills during the rehearsals! The tests with sleeping pills are carried out separately as described above - it is only about testing your reaction to the medication. Do not practice in combination with sleeping pills and plastic bag! Since you choose a large bag that allows you to breathe for about 50 minutes, it is not dangerous to pull the bag over your head (without taking any medication) and try out how it works with the attachment under the elastic band. So swing the bag through the air to fill it, lie down or sit down and place the bag on your head. Can the ends be fixed under the rubber band so that no surrounding air can enter? Experiment with whether it is comfortable to wear a wide-brimmed hat. How does it work with the hat when you are lying down (if this is your preferred position)? You should practice the procedure so that you know exactly what to do when you actually do it. Remember that it is possible that your ability to act may be limited by an illness if you actually want to carry out the suicide. In addition to this, you will have taken a large amount of sleeping pills beforehand when doing the "real" procedure and these pills may work very quickly. You must be finished with the preparations and already lie in the intended position (or sit well fixed) before the sleeping pill takes effect. So there is not much time left for you to try things out during the actual procedure - all remaining questions should be clarified beforehand.

Now, when the day of the actual execution has come, start taking the antiemetic according to the schedule described above. According to this schedule, you should start taking the antiemetic 24 hours before the planned suicide; the last dose is taken 45 minutes before the sedative. If it is an emergency situation that requires a quick implementation, you can also split the recommended dose of the antiemetic between the last two doses. Do not eat a large meal on the day of your planned suicide. A light meal (for example one or two slices of toast) is well suited. Make sure that you are undisturbed for at least two hours, preferably longer. Get everything ready. The place where you want to lie (or sit) should be completely prepared. Then take the sedatives. You can either powder or crush them in advance and stir them into a small bowl of applesauce or similar, which you spoon out quickly, or you swallow the tablets as they are. It is basically not such a large amount of tablets that pulverization is necessary, but some people have problems with swallowing in general or swallowing tablets, so the intake of pulverized or crushed tablets is of course possible. However, remember that the effect of powdered or crushed tablets is faster, as the active ingredient can be absorbed by the body more quickly. You can also drink some alcohol after taking the sedatives - a glass of wine, for example. Do not drink alcohol that you are not used to and do not drink large quantities. In the worst case, this could mean that you will vomit despite having taken the antiemetic beforehand, which would put the success of the procedure at risk.

After taking the sleeping pills, place the elastic bands around your neck (ideally above or below the larynx). The rubber bands should be close to your neck but not uncomfortable. Swing the bag once around the room so that it opens and fills with air inside. Then place the bag on your head and fasten the ends securely under the rubber bands. You can also turn on your favourite music or insert a meditation CD, a dream journey or similar. Then move into the prepared position and wait for the sleeping pills to take effect.

In case you have previously made arrangements with someone to remove the plastic bag from your head after successful self-determined dying in order to hide the cause of death and make the death look "natural", it is important to make sure that this is not done too early. In some cases it was wrongly assumed that death had already occurred and the suicide failed because the plastic bag was removed too early by a second person. In the context of wanting to maintain a visually positive impression after death, I would also like to point out that during death there is a loosening of the sphincter muscles and thus a discharge of faeces and urine.

CPSIA information can be obtained
at www.ICGtesting.com
Printed in the USA
LVHW092058210322
714007LV00007B/940